Low Back & Leg Pain:
What It Is and How It Is Treated

Contents
5	The Spine
6-7	The Normal Disc
8-9	Disc Degeneration & Arthritis
10-11	Disc Injuries
12-14	Sciatica
14-16	Treatment of the Disc
17	Movements to Avoid
18-19	Facet Syndrome
20	Short Leg
21	Sprain / Strain
21	Vertebral Subluxation
22	Spondylolisthesis
23	Sacroiliac Subluxation
23	Tropism
24	Scoliosis
25	Transitional Vertebra
26-27	Stenosis
28	The Pregnant Patient with Back and/or Leg Pain
29	Post-Surgical Continued Pain—Back Pain and/or Leg Pain
30-32	Treatment of Low Back Pain
33-34	Care Instructions
35	About the author

> *Dear Patient:*
>
> Your condition and its care are described on page(s) _____. Please read it carefully. Have your spouse or a friend read it also to help you in your care and recovery.

Introduction

The low back pain or leg pain you are experiencing can be very disturbing to your lifestyle. It may prevent work and play; sitting, riding, or even walking. You may feel frustrated over the recurrence of pain. People have trouble understanding why they have back pain and, even more, why it does not always totally resolve. For some patients, control of pain rather than cure is the goal.

This book is written to help you understand the common causes of low back pain which are basically two: one is a disc condition in which sprain or tearing of the elastic fibers of the disc cause pain and sometimes allow swelling of the disc to compress a nerve and result in leg pain called sciatica, and the other cause is joint irritation at the motion areas of one vertebra with another. Each of these conditions will be discussed in this book and your doctor will direct you to the findings that seem to be causing your low back or leg pain.

Chiropractic care is reportedly *used by over 50% of Americans for their low back pain.* The Agency for Health Care Policy and Research of the U.S. Department of Health and Human Services cited spinal manipulation as a top effective treatment for low back pain. Doctors of Chiropractic devote their academic years of professional education and subsequent internship to the study and care of spinal conditions and back pain. We are sensitive to your spinal pain and are specially trained in its diagnosis and treatment. Even after graduation, some continue to study for specialty certification in the care of low back pain conditions.

Surgery is necessary for less than 2% of low back pain patients. At least 6 to 8 weeks of active, non-surgical care (chiropractic) should be given before surgery is considered, unless neurological problems as urination difficulties or progressive muscle weakening occur.

Your Doctor of Chiropractic cooperates with other health care professionals to ensure that you receive the best care possible. Your chiropractor may instruct you in the home care of your back problem to aid healing and to prevent recurrence. He or she may also invite you to a low back wellness school which will show you how to perform your activities of daily living without causing pain. Nutritional factors in the care of your spine can be helpful.

Note: Throughout this book, outcomes from a collection of data from a 1000 patient cases study [*Topics in Clinical Chiropractic* 1996; 3(3)] are referenced for the number of days and number of visits for the patients to attain maximum improvement under this form of care. The results, diagnosis notwithstanding, are that (1) less than 90 days were needed to attain maximum improvement for 91% of patients, (2) the average number of days to maximum improvement was 30, and (3) the average number of visits was 12.

Two basic sources of low back pain are agreed upon by most authorities: the intervertebral disc and the articular facets. These sources and their causes of pain follow.

THE SPINE

The spine has 4 curves or sections: *cervical, thoracic, lumbar,* and *sacral.* As the old saying goes, "stand up straight." This keeps your spine's curves balanced in order to support you when you move. An aligned spine lessens the chance of injury and stress on the spine.

The spine is composed of:
— vertebrae (the bones of the spine),
— intervertebral discs (the spongy pads separating the vertebrae),
— the spinal cord,
— spinal nerves,
— articular facet joints, and
— the sacrum. (Figure 1)

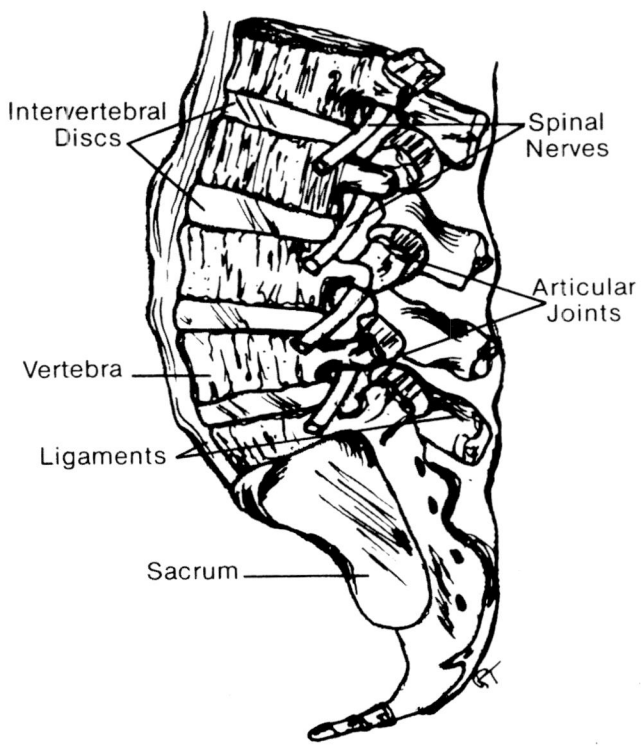

Figure 1

THE DISC

Normal

The intervertebral disc separates the vertebrae (bones) of the spine and cushions them like a shock absorber. The center of the disc (nucleus pulposus) is a gel-like material contained by the anular fibers, sensitive pain fibers which circle and contain the nucleus like rubberbands. The vertebra above balances over the nucleus and depends on it for spinal movement. (Figure 2)

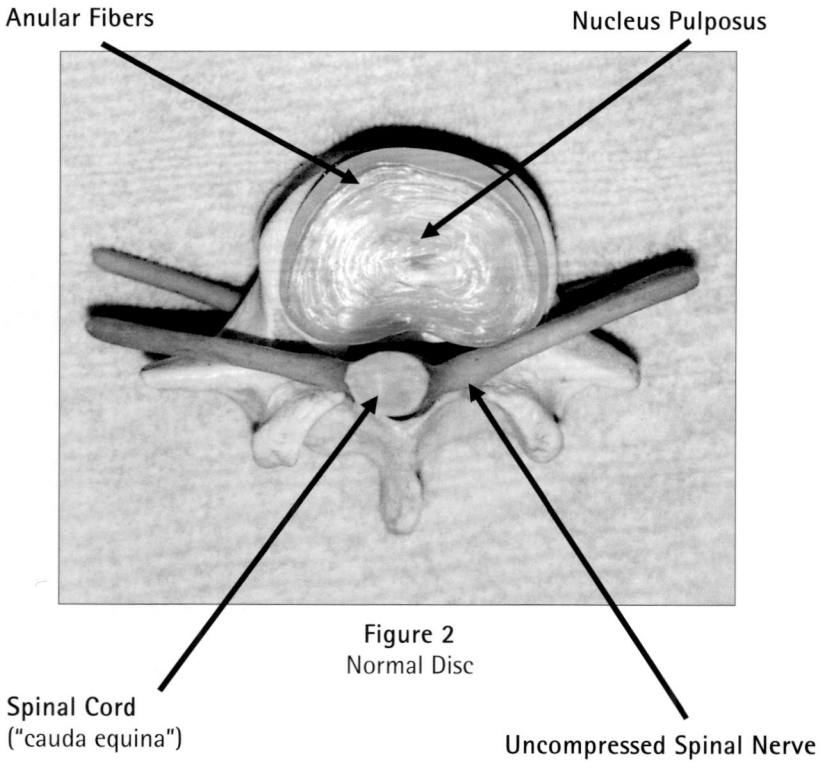

Figure 2
Normal Disc

On MRI, the back of the disc is smooth and not protruding into the spinal cord. The curved arrow shows the nerve exiting from the spinal cord when it is not compressed by disc herniation material (straight arrow). (Figure 3)

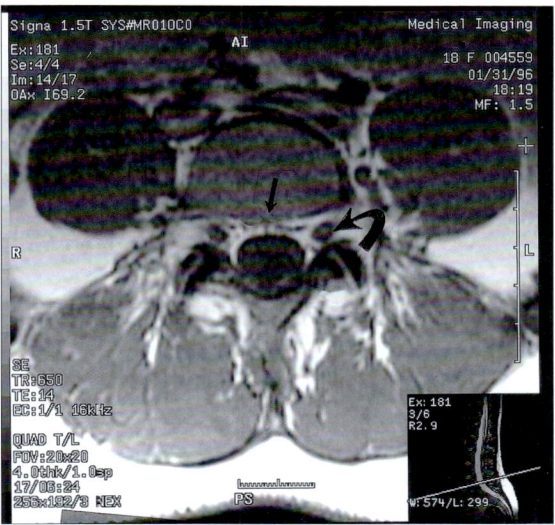

Figure 3

The intervertebral disc is a spongy pad which holds the *vertebrae* (bones) of the spine apart. (See arrow in Figure 4.) The *disc* separates and cushions the movement of the vertebrae. A normal disc gives a large space between the vertebrae as seen in the x-ray.

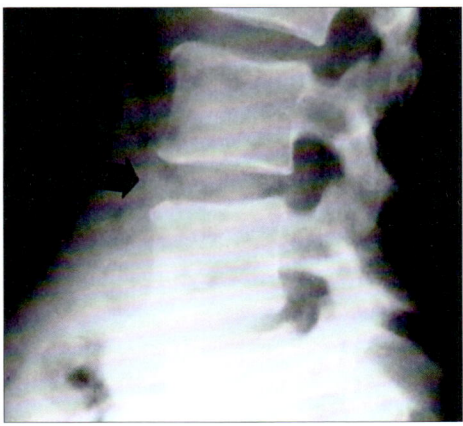

Figure 4

Abnormalities of the Disc

Disc Degeneration

A disc becomes *abnormal* when it loses its nucleus' fluid due to degeneration (nutrition loss) or injury or arthritis. Such problems produce pain by disc space thinning (Figure 5A - a condition called ***disc degeneration***), facet articulation misalignment (Figure 5B - a condition called ***subluxation***), and spinal nerve opening reduction (Figure 5C — a condition termed ***stenosis***). This compression can result in pain in the low back and/or pain down the leg (*sciatica*).

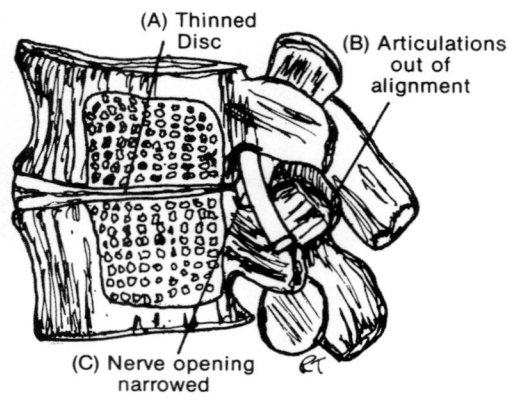

Figure 5 (A, B, C)

Disc degeneration can be seen on x-ray. Figure 5D shows a degenerated L5 disc (see small arrow) and its smaller nerve opening (outlined in a white, broken line) compared to the normal disc (see large arrow) and its larger nerve opening (see its white, broken line).

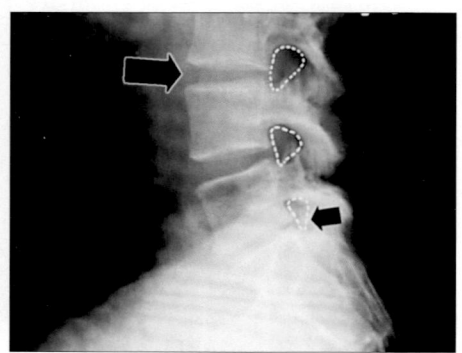

Figure 5D

When the degeneration progresses, *bone spurs (claw spurs)* develop on the vertebrae. (Figure 6)

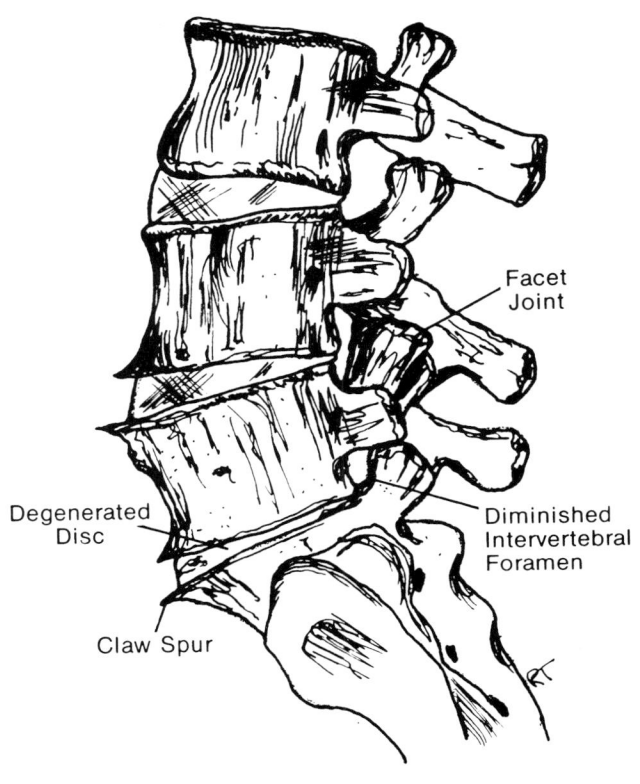

Figure 6

ARTHRITIS

A note on *"arthritis"* as a diagnosis of low back pain: arthritis is *not* always a cause of pain. Further it is misleading to say the *only* reason for a person's low back or leg pain is arthritis.

Disc Injuries

- a *ruptured* or *herniated* or *extruded disc* – the nucleus pushes *through* the anular fibers of the disc and leaks into the spinal canal, irritating the spinal nerves with pressure or with a chemical reaction
- a *bulging, protruding* or *slipped disc* - the nucleus pushes *on* the anular fibers of the disc, pressing on the spinal nerves

When a disc's nucleus pulposus loses its fluidity, the spine moves abnormally. Any tearing or ripping of the disc may result in shifting of the gel-like substance of this nucleus backward and gradually putting pressure against ("pinching") the sciatic nerve roots. (Figures 7 and 8)

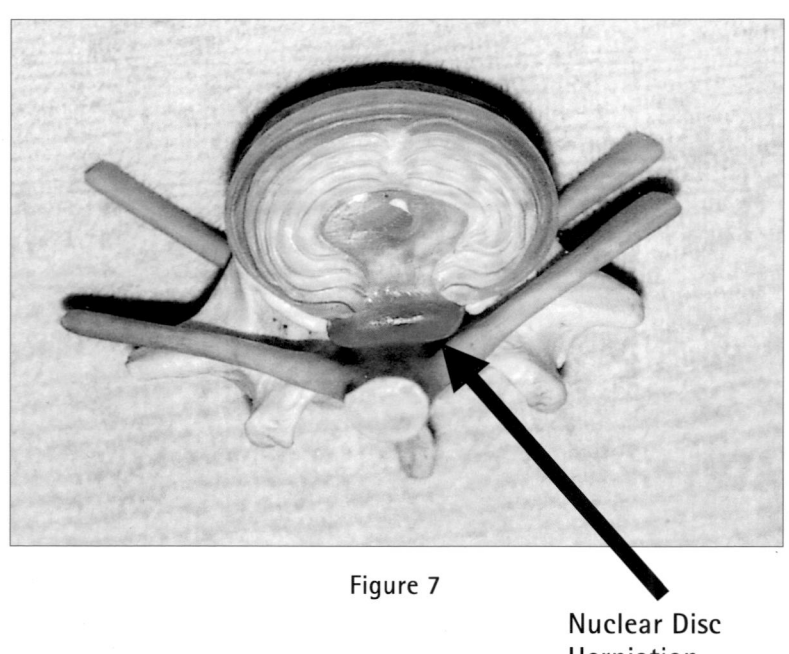

Figure 7

Nuclear Disc Herniation

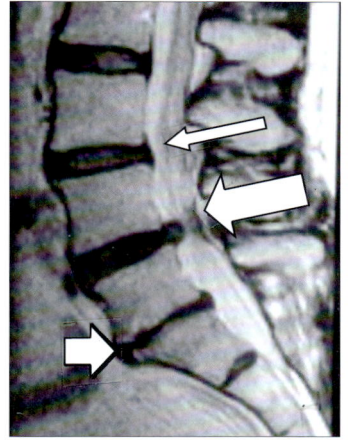

Figure 8a

Figure 8a
This MRI side view shows a large disc herniation (middle white arrowhead), normal disc (top arrowhead), and a degenerated disc (bottom arrowhead).

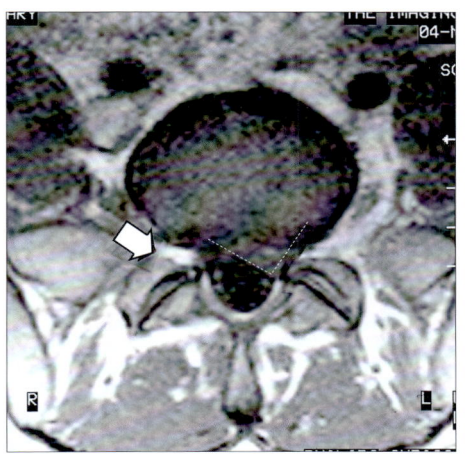

Figure 8b

Figure 8b
This MRI view looks down on the spine and shows the large disc herniation (outlined in white broken line). Note the normal nerve space on the opposite side (white arrowhead) where the disc is not herniated.

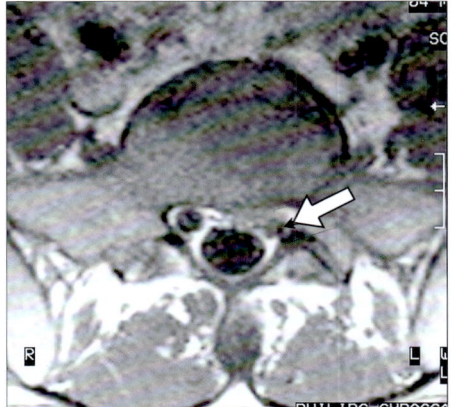

Figure 8c

Figure 8c
Note on this MRI image that the nerve (white arrow) is engulfed with disc herniation material. Compare this to the normal nerve visible on the left.

SCIATICA

Leg pain is referred to as SCIATICA.

The slipping of the nucleus will result in back pain and, possibly, pain down the leg (*sciatica*). The amount of pain depends upon the severity of the disc slippage or rupture. The more pressure from the disc on the nerve, the further down the leg the pain will go. (Figure 9)

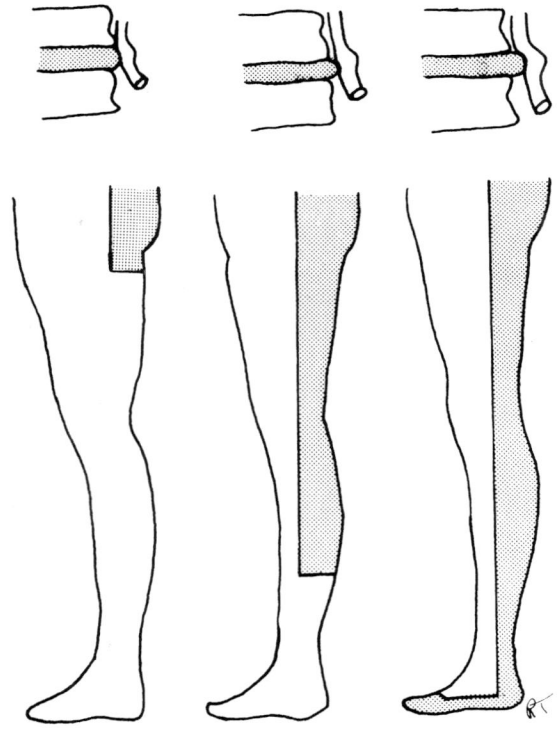

Figure 9

Sciatic pain distribution varies according to which nerve root is compressed by a disc bulge, herniation, slip, protrusion.

The location of the pain in the leg indicates which sciatic nerve root is compressed. (Figures 10a, b, c)

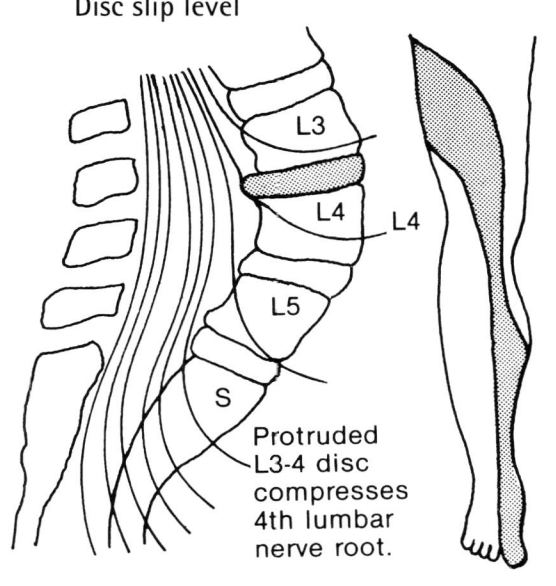

Figure 10a

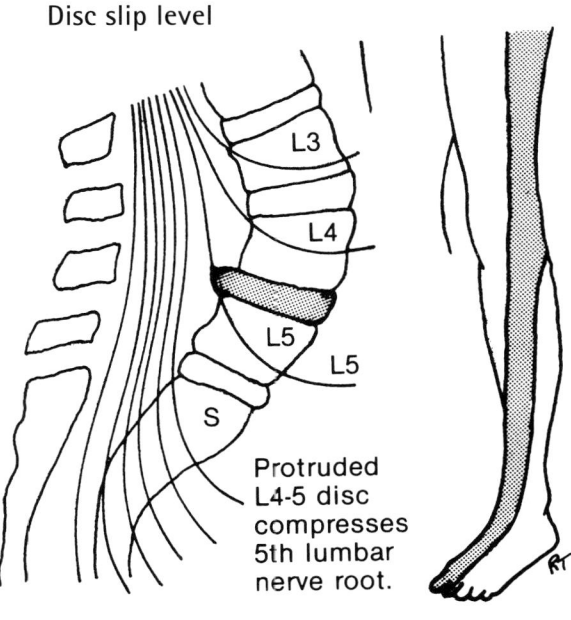

Figure 10b

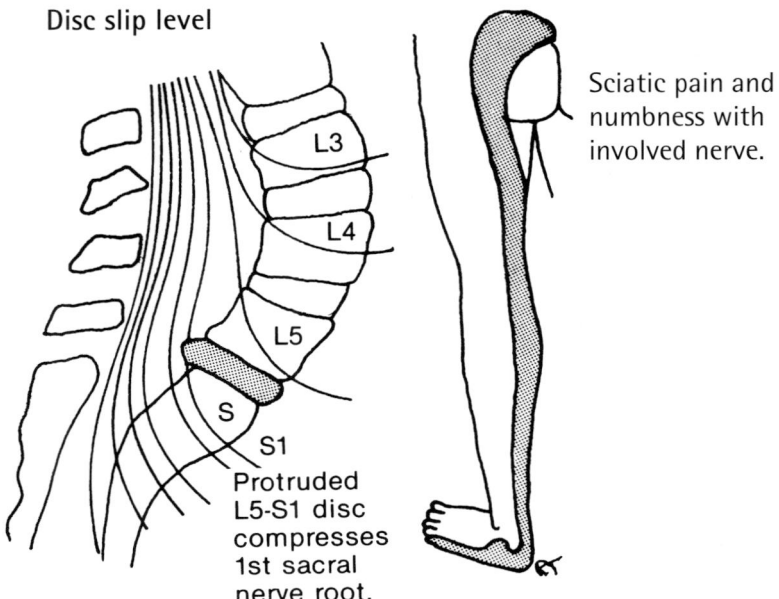

Figure 10c

Bending, lifting, twisting -- worsens the pain when a disc has slipped. (See page 10.) The pain is usually in one leg. It may range from a dull ache to a sharp stabbing pain extending from the back to the foot. The pain may be described as burning, numb, pins and needles, "worms crawling in the skin," tingling. Severe cases may even result in the inability to move the leg.

Treatment of the Disc:

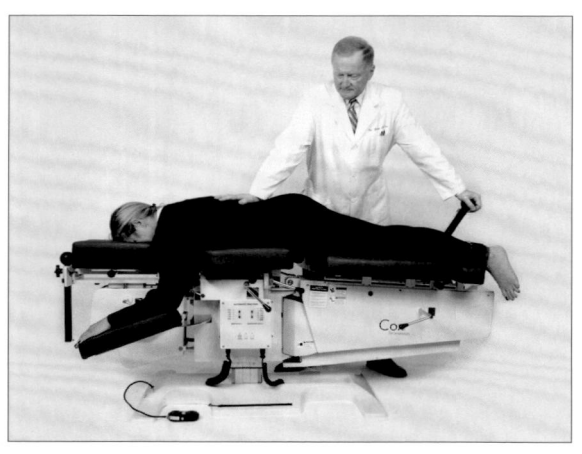

Figure 11

Cox® flexion-distraction and decompression manipulation is applied to the lumbar spine (Figure 11) to bring about the change shown in Figure 12. This non-surgical care is commonly accepted in treating disc problems before resorting to surgery.

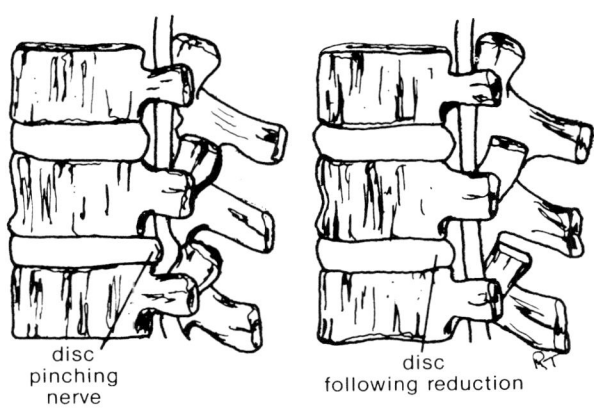

Figure 12

With a disc problem, you may be treated more often in the beginning of care at the doctor's office. As you improve, your visits will be cut. The "rule of 50%" is observed:

The 50% Rule for Care and Referral

At 50% improvement, the frequency of treatments is reduced by 50%. If you do not attain 50% improvement and relief of pain within a month of care, further tests like MRI or CT scans may be ordered to study your spine in more detail. Depending on these tests' outcomes, surgery may be considered. If at any time signs of progression of the condition are noted, a referral will be made.

This intensive treatment regime allows healing to proceed without the irritating movements like sitting, bending, twisting, etc., that hinder and hurt the body's attempt to heal.

Length of Care:

It takes three months for a torn disc to heal well enough to allow you to return to daily activities: prolonged sitting, lifting, twisting, etc. The first 3 to 4 weeks of concentrated treatment and therapies are designed to allow the best opportunity for the disc to heal quickly.

Clinical Outcomes in Patients with Disc Herniation:
Less than 90 days to maximum improvement: 91% of patients
Less than 30 visits to maximum improvement: 70% of patients

TREATMENT RESPONSIBILITIES FOR DISC PATIENTS:

Doctor's:
— lower the pressure inside the disc so the nucleus returns to the center of the disc with distraction adjustments
— aid in the healing of the torn anular fibers of the disc
— drive out the chemicals that irritate and inflame the spinal nerves

Yours:
— Follow *all* the guidelines suggested on pages 33-34, especially these:
    — Do not sit.
    — Wear a support brace as/if directed. It assures a quick heal.
    — Take a glucosamine sulfate/chondroitin sulfate supplement, like Discat Plus.
    — Avoid constipation!
    — Get a good supportive chair and mattress.
    — Modify your daily activities and work, as necessary.

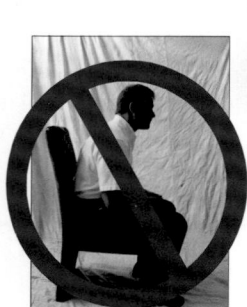
Don't sit.

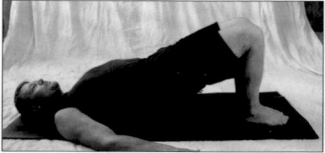
Exercise.

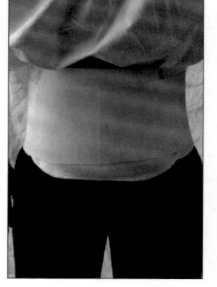
Wear back support.

Special Note on *Sciatica* As You Heal:

It is important to realize the seriousness of sciatic pain. It is discouraging when you get along fine and then feel that old pain start back again. Please know that this may be expected. *It is common to have recurrences during healing.* Study the movements below that lead to or irritate low back and sciatic pain and those that may help you avoid pain.

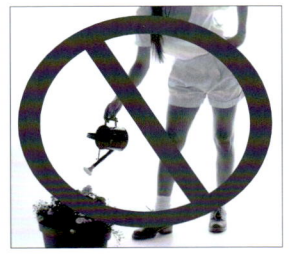

Don't bend and twist at the same time!

Keep the vacuum sweeper (rake, shovel, etc.) *in front of you.*

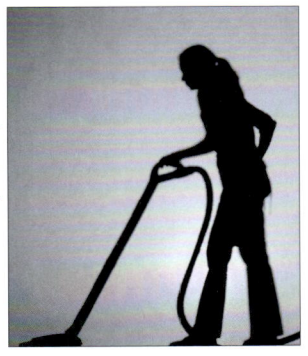

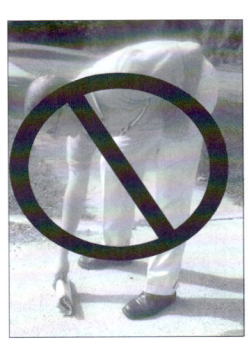

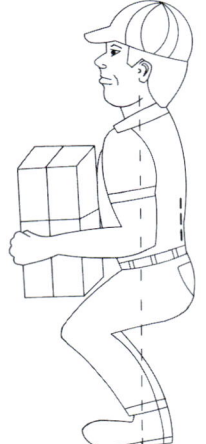

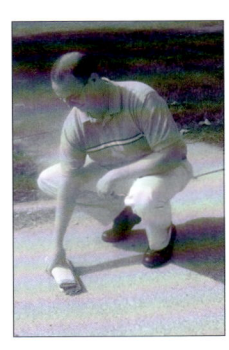

Don't bend and lift together!
Instead, lift with the object as close to your
body as possible, tighten abdomen,
keep hips forward.
Use your knees.

Other Spinal Abnormalities Causing Low Back Pain

Facet Syndrome

- affects 26% of people with low back pain.
- is a common condition.
- is a misalignment of one vertebra with the vertebra adjacent to it because the disc is narrowed at the back and widened at the front. (Figure 13)
- is painful as the spinal nerve root is compressed, the facet and disc are irritated. *All are pain producing.*

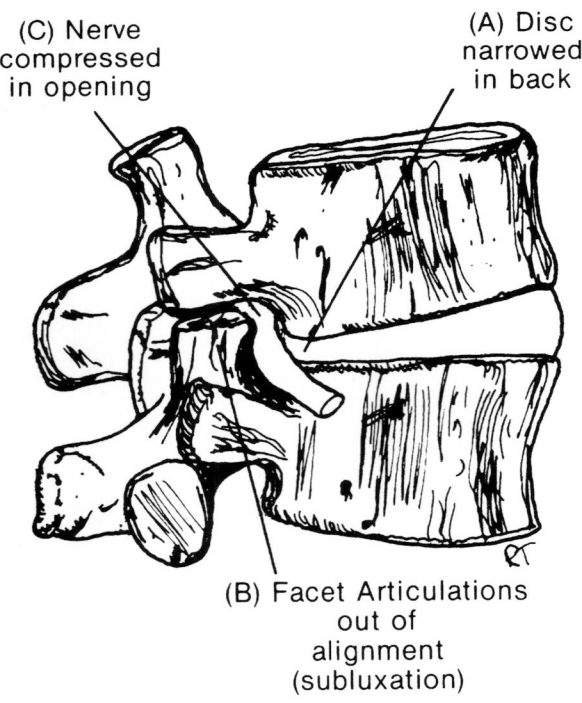

(C) Nerve compressed in opening

(A) Disc narrowed in back

(B) Facet Articulations out of alignment (subluxation)

Figure 13

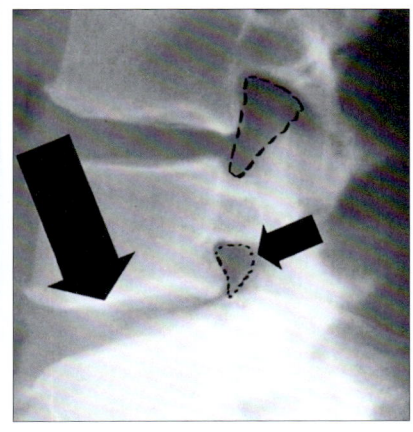 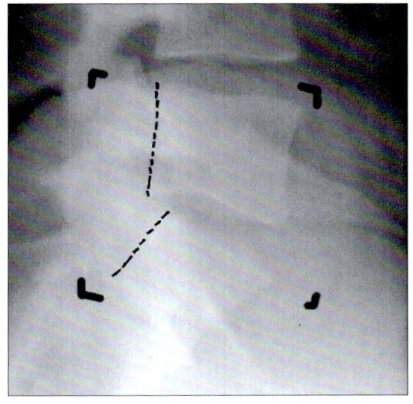

Figure 14

Figure 15
Retrolisthesis Subluxation

The large arrow in Figure 14 shows the narrowed disc. The small arrow shows the minimized nerve opening. The level above this is normal.

Figure 15 shows retrolisthesis subluxation, a backward movement of a vertebra on the vertebra below, caused by instability of the disc, disc degeneration, and muscle weakness.

As people grow older, their ciscs lose water and shrink in height. Further, they allow their abdominal and low back muscles to weaken. All of this results in narrowing of the disc space and nerve opening, thus trapping the nerve so it becomes painful.

Clinical Outcomes in Patients with Facet Syndrome:
Less than 90 days to maximum improvement: 90% of patients
Less than 30 visits to maximum improvement: 81% of patients

Treatment Responsibilities for Facet Syndrome:

Doctor's:
— Open the nerve opening.
— Increase the disc space.
— Realign the vertebrae and facet joints.

Yours:
— Perform the recommended specific exercises.
— Avoid certain movements that are bad for your back. (See page 17.)
— Bend and lift properly.
— Follow marked instructions on pages 33-34.

Short Leg

— affects 11% of people

Having a short leg is like driving a car with two different sized tires on the rear axle. These x-rays show a patient with a short leg (Figure 16) and the same patient with a shoe build-up to correct the problem (Figure 17).

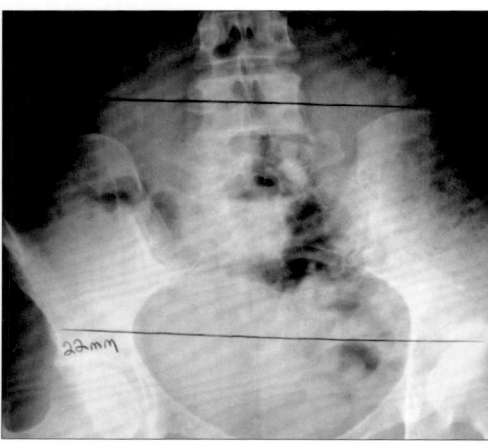

Figure 16

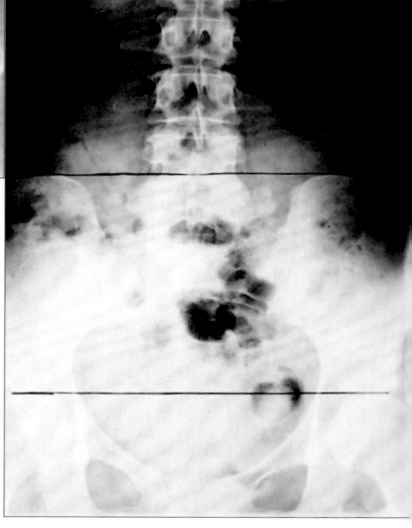

Figure 17

Treatment Responsibilities for Short Leg:

Doctor's:
— Correct the difference in leg lengths.
— Align your spine with manipulation.

Yours:
— Wear the foot or heel orthotics customized for you *all the time.*

Sprain / Strain Injury

— muscle stretch and tearing
— after vehicle accidents, falls, lifting, etc.

Sprain/strain injuries can require 4 to 16 weeks to heal.

Vertebral Subluxation

— misalignment of one vertebra upon another

On this x-ray, one vertebra is tilted to the right (arrows). This results in irritation of the soft tissues and nerves at this level leading to low back and maybe even some leg pain. (Figure 18)

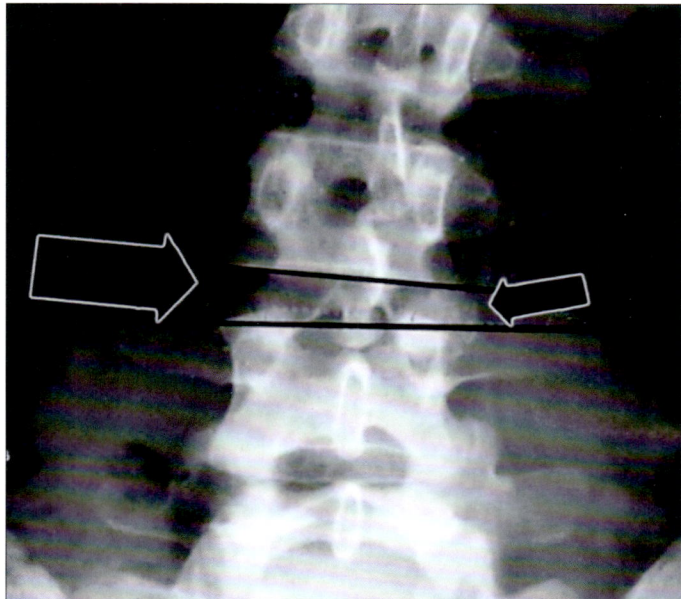

Figure 18

Spondylolisthesis

- affects 6% of people, usually at the 5th lumbar level
- usually evolves early in life due to failure of strong bone formation in the vertebra
- is most serious in teens, especially if symptoms persist or worsen
- also occurs with disc degeneration and spinal arthritis

Spondylolisthesis stems from a fracture in the middle of the vertebra which allows the front part of one vertebra (Figure 19 - small arrow) to slip forward on the vertebra below (Figure 19 - large arrow). The fracture is called a "stress" fracture due to repeated stresses applied to a weakened area of bone by contact sports like football, hockey, etc.

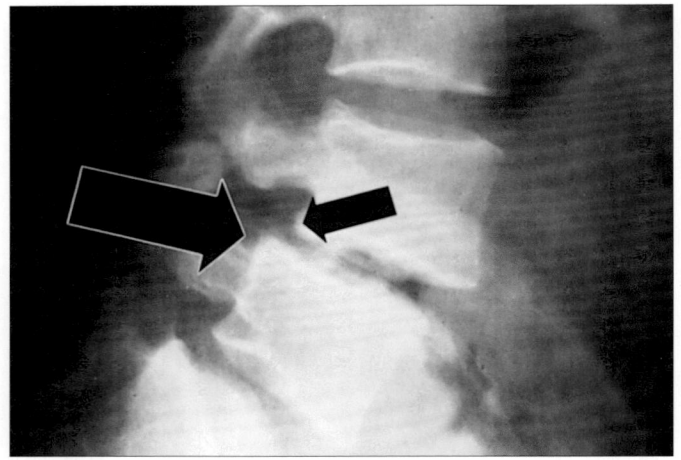

Figure 19

Outcomes:
Less than 90 days to maximum improvement: 95% of patients
Less than 30 visits to maximum improvement: 90% of patients

Treatment Responsibilities for Spondylolisthesis:

Doctor's:
- Adjust the spine to reduce the stress created by slippage of the vertebrae.

Yours:
- Follow instructions on pages 33-34.

Sacroiliac Subluxation

The sacroiliac joints can be a cause of pain. They are shown at the arrows in Figure 20. Manipulation can relieve this pain.

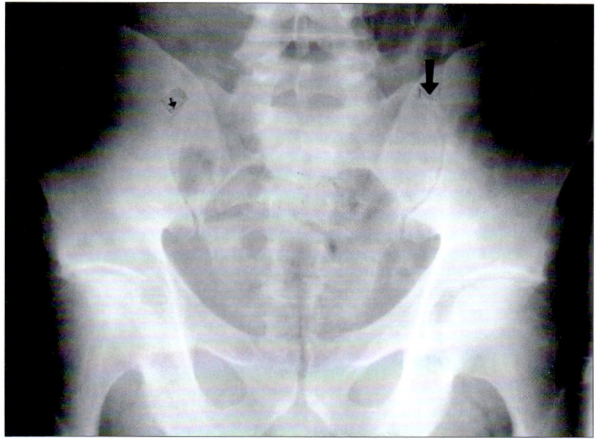

Figure 20

Tropism

Tropism is a developmental abnormality of facet orientation which leads to increased disc stress. In tropism, the joints (arrows in Figure 21) are faced differently. They only move with great stress. This may lead to disc degeneration and/or disc herniation.

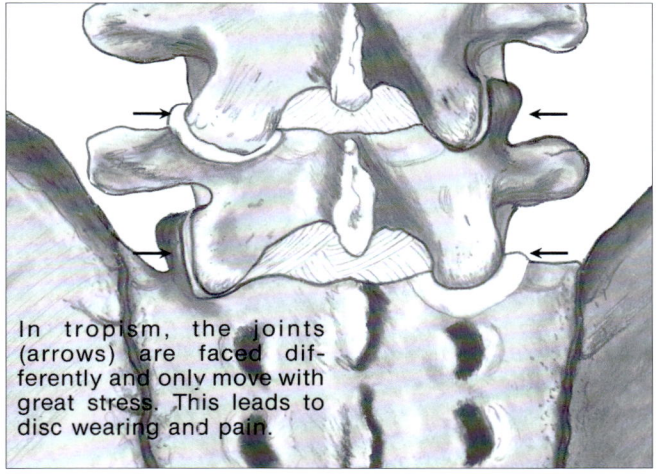

Figure 21

Scoliosis

- affects 10% of people
- occurs 7 times more often in girls than in boys
- is hereditary
- is noticeable during teenage years when growth is rapid
- is a deviation of spinal curvature producing body disfigurement (Figure 22)
- is referred to as "idiopathic" as it has no known cause
- may have a nutritional deficiency component

Scoliosis can stop its progressive curvature or continue through life. Your physician will identify and thus monitor the progress of scoliosis. In addition to monitoring your condition, your physician may recommend exercises, manipulation, bracing, even surgery in certain cases.

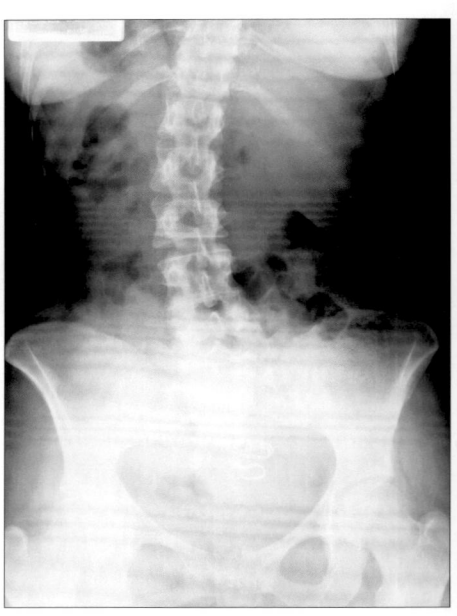

Figure 22

Treatment Responsibilities for Scoliosis:

Doctor's:
- Adjust the spine to allow easier and pain-free mobility.
- Carefully monitor the progression of the curve.

Yours:
- Keep doctor appointments.
- Wear a special brace as/if prescribed.
- Perform exercises as prescribed.
- Follow nutritional advice—*important.*

Transitional Vertebra

- affects 6% of people
- is a congenital anomaly
- causes instability of the spine
- stresses the low back
- one too many or one too few lumbar vertebrae (6 or 4 vertebrae, respectively) instead of the usual 5 (Figures 23 and 24)

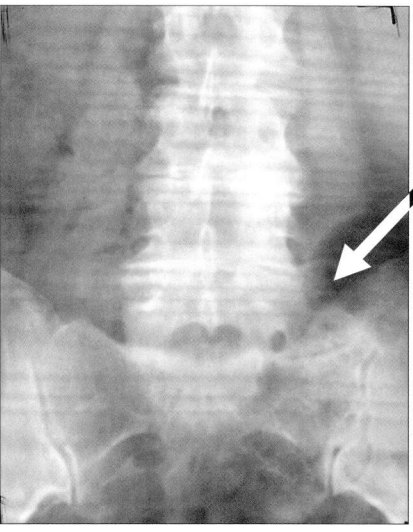

Figure 23

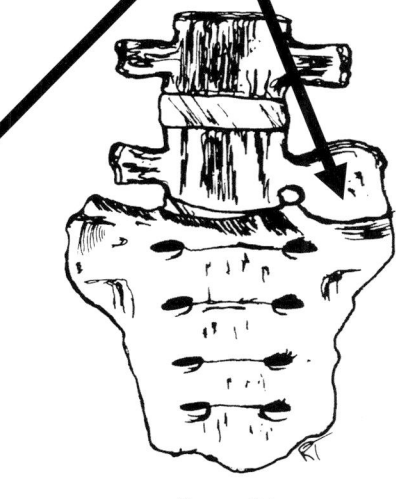

Overdeveloped transverse process causing transitional vertebra

Figure 24

In a recent research study, this condition proved to require more treatments and days to attain relief than any other problem in the low back. Therefore, you need to follow your doctor's directions carefully.

Outcomes:
Less than 90 days to maximum improvement: 93% of patients
Less than 30 visits to maximum improvement: 94% of patients

Treatment Responsibilities for Transitional Segment:

Doctor's:
- Use the specific chiropractic adjustment for this condition.

Yours:
- Follow instructions on pages 33-34.

Stenosis

— the narrowing of any natural body opening -- In the spine, the narrowing of the spinal canal opening is of concern.

In the normal spine, the spinal canal is wide with abundant space for the spinal cord and its exiting nerves. (top left drawing of Figure 25; Figure 26) In a stenotic canal, there is a small opening though which the cord *and* its nerves must pass. (See Figure 25 and 27.) Since the canal is small, the nerves are compressed.

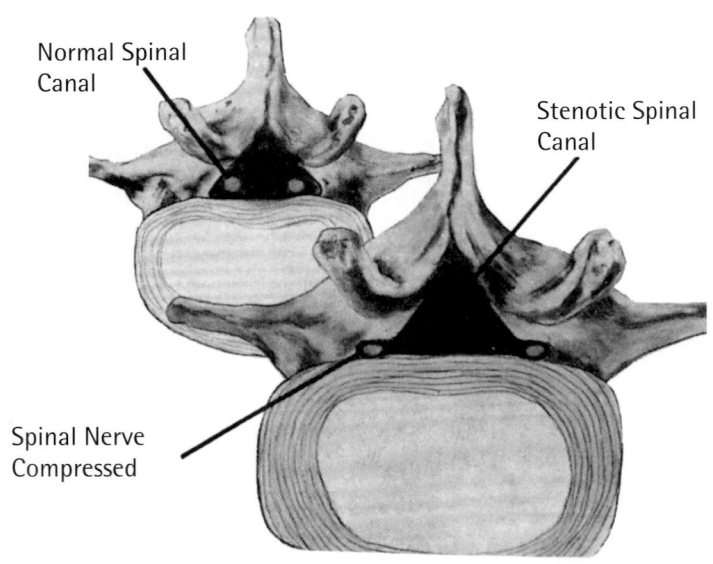

Figure 25

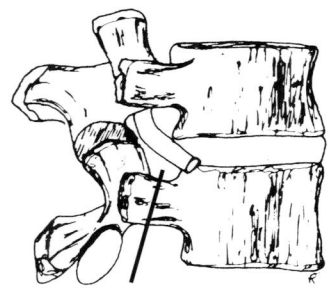

Normal Nerve Opening

Figure 26

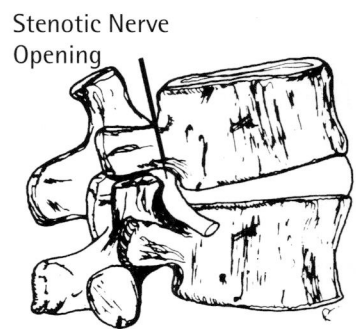

Figure 27

The MRI of a normal spinal canal shows a wide opening for the spinal cord and nerves. (Figure 28 – See arrows.)

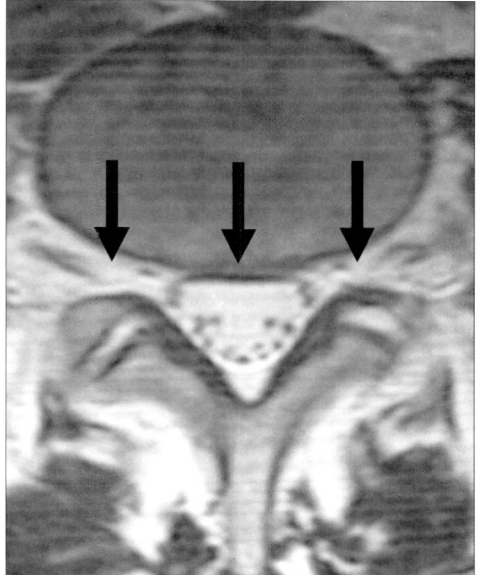

Figure 28

The MRI of a stenotic spinal canal shows decreased space for the spinal cord and nerves. (Figure 29—See arrows.)

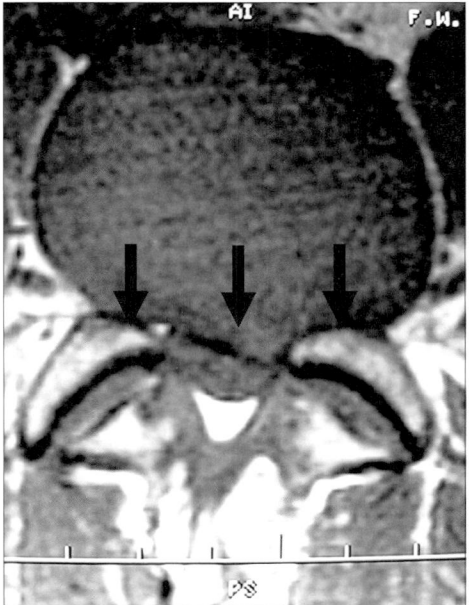

Figure 29

The Pregnant Patient with Back and/or Leg Pain

Low back pain occurs in *61% of pregnant women* but only 25% of providers recommend treatment. *Chiropractic adjustments relieved 94% of pregnant women's low back pain within 4.5 days with two treatments.* No adverse effects were reported. Chiropractic is suggested to be safe and effective in reducing low back pain intensity in pregnant women. (1)

In another study, *69% of pregnant women* reported low back pain during pregnancy. **Risk factors** for it were (a) younger age and (b) a history of low back pain without pregnancy or with a previous pregnancy. The pain caused sleep disturbance and impaired daily living due to pain. (2)

Chiropractic adjustment using Cox® flexion-distraction treatment relieved back pain in a 26 year old pregnant woman with pain radiating down the leg *in just one visit.* Complete resolution of symptoms was noted in 8 visits. Due to the special condition of the patient, she is placed in a special position (side-lying with the belly to the physician) for the treatment. (See Figure 30.) (3)

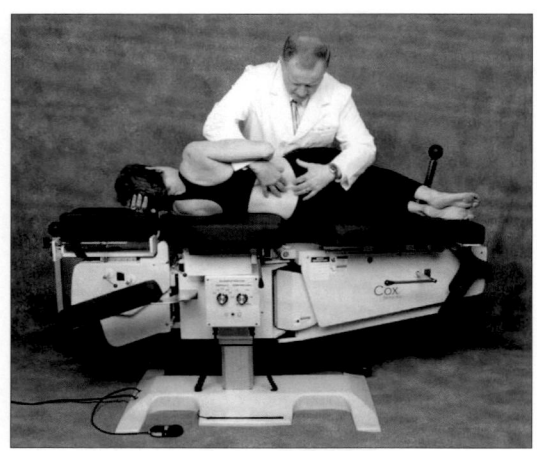

Figure 30
special position for treating pregnant patients as well as patients who are uncomfortable or unable to lie on the stomach

References:
1. Lisi AJ: Chiropractic spinal manipulation for low back pain of pregnancy: a retrospective case series. J Midwidery Womens Health 2006; 51(1):e7-10
2. Wang SM, Dezinno P, Maranets I, Berman MR, Caldwell-Andews AA, Kain ZN: Low back pain during pregnancy: prevalence, risk factors, and outcomes. Obstet Gynecol 2004; 104(1):65-70
3. Kruse RA, Gudavalli SR, Cambron J: Chiropractic treatment of a pregnant patient with radiculopathy. J of Chiropractic Medicine 2007; 6(4):153-158

The Post-Surgical Continued Pain Patient with Low Back and/or Leg Pain

Post-surgical continued pain (*formerly called failed back surgery syndrome*) is defined by the International Association for the Study of Pain (IASP) as "*lumbar spinal pain of unknown origin, either persisting despite surgical intervention or appearing after surgical intervention*". (1)

In the United States, more low back surgeries are performed per capita than in any other country. (2) Half of spine surgery patients are improved, and half are the same or worse one year later. (3)

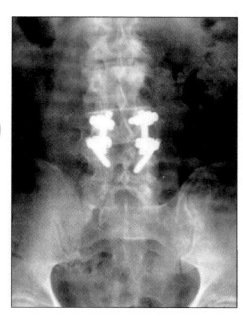

Pre-Surgery Care
Studies recommend spinal manipulation as a pre-surgical treatment plan for back and radicular patients.
- A trial of conservative non-operative care is advised before surgery for patients with lumbar disc herniation. (4)
- Non-surgical rehabilitation of chronic low back patients showed equal benefit to surgery in relieving pain. Further, surgery was more costly, carried a potential risk and was not cost-effective. (5)
- First-time lumbar disc surgery rates drop by nearly two-thirds when sciatica patients with and without low back pain were treated non-surgically in a multidisciplinary spine clinic. (6)
- 76% pain improvement and 73% disability improvement is reported in lumbar spinal stenosis patients treated with Cox® distraction and/or neural mobilization. (7)

Cox® Technic for Post-Surgery Care
In a study of 32 post-surgical patients, some with fusion and some without, who had continued pain and sought chiropractic care, a 41% drop in pain is reported overall. Patients who had fusion report a 57% drop in pain. Best of all, no adverse side effects are reported. (8) Further, a patient treated for post-surgical bi-lateral leg pain and low back pain found 100% leg pain relief and 70% back pain relief in 20 visits in 3 months. (9)

References:
1. Evans RC: Failed back surgery syndrome: definition, etiology and diagnostic evaluation. Lecture presentation, Amer College of Chiro Orthopedists Conference Proceedings. Investigation of Failed Back Surgery. Hyatt Regency, San Antonio May 2009:1-28
2. Cherkin, DC, Deyo RA: An international comparison of back surgery rates. Spine 1994;19(11);1201-6
3. Haugen, AJ; Grovle, L; Brox, JI. Estimates of success in patients with sciatica due to lumbar disc herniation depend upon outcome measure. European Spine Journal 2011;20 (10):1669-1675
4. Daffner SD, Hymanson HJ, Wang JC: Cost and use of conservative management of lumbar disc herniation before surgical discectomy. Spine Journal 2010;10 (6)463-468
5. Fairbank J et al: Randomized controlled trial to compare surgical stabilization of the lumbar spine with an intensive rehabilitation program for patients with chronic low back pain. The MRC stabilization trial. British Med J 2005;330(7502):1233-39
6. Rasmussen C et al: Rates of lumbar disc surgery before and after implementation of multidisciplinary nonsurgical spine clinics. Spine.2005; 30(21):2469-73
7. Murphy DR et al: A non-surgical approach to the management of lumbar spinal stenosis: A prospective observational cohort study. BMC Musculoskeletal Disorders 7. Feb 23 2006. p.nil_1-nil_8
8. Kruse R, Cambron J: Chiropractic Management of Postsurgical Lumbar Spine Pain: A Retrospective Study of 32 Cases. JMPT 2011; 34(6):408-12
9. Cox JM in reference 1.

TREATMENT of
LOW BACK & LEG PAIN *

The success or failure in correcting your problem conservatively rests largely with you. It is commonly accepted that even in treating patients with slipped discs, out-patient, conservative, aggressive management should be tried before resorting to surgery. The potential complications related to surgery, the certainty that such will cause damage to the stability of the spine, and the occasional failure of surgical procedures to relieve symptoms indicate the advisability of a serious conservative treatment regime first.

You will be expected to follow the guidelines set forth to help your spine heal. The only one hurt by not following such guidelines is you, the patient.

1. For the first three weeks, you may be instructed to come in for treatment every day if you have low back and leg pain. If you respond more quickly, the treatments will be less frequent according to the "rule of 50%" as described on page 15. For maximum results in, be prepared to come in daily for the first three weeks if you have disc herniation causing sciatica or leg pain. Treatment may be given more than once a day for severe pain.

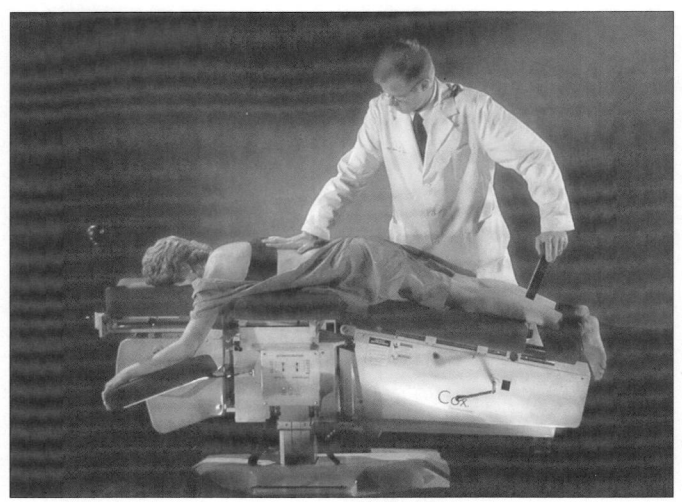

Figure 31
Treatment for facet syndrome and spondylolisthesis

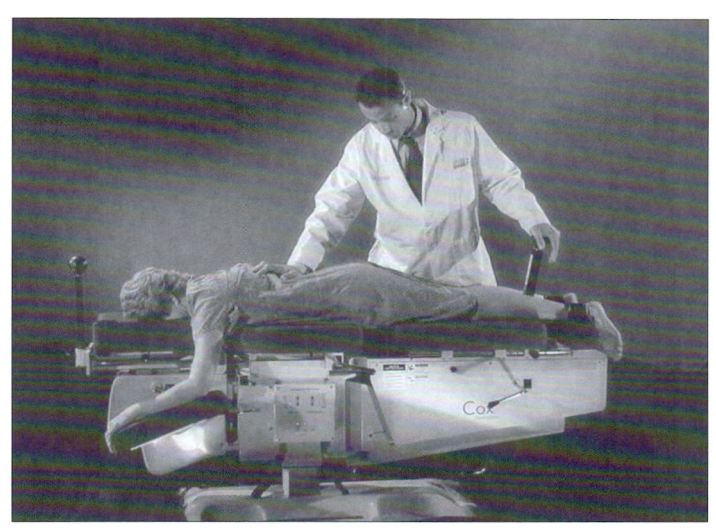

Figure 32
Treatment for disc protrusion, subluxation, scoliosis, arthritis, transitional vertebra

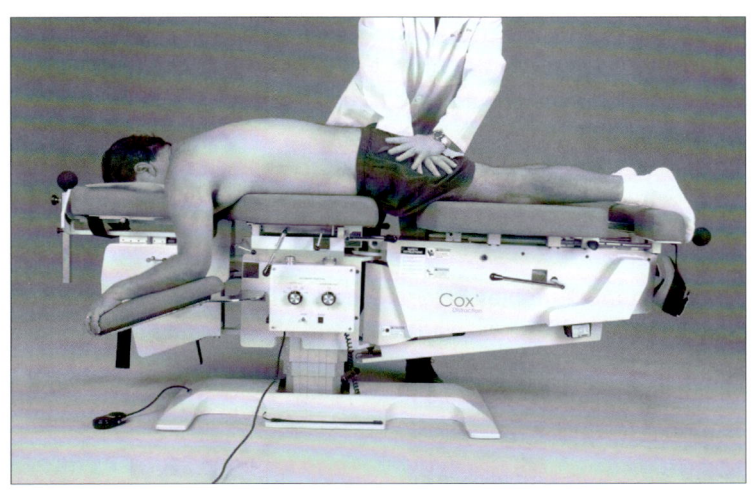

Figure 33
Treatment for sacroiliac pain

2. Physical therapy will be applied to your spine to ease pain, help remove the swelling that accompanies the problems, and relieve muscle spasm. (See Figure 34.)

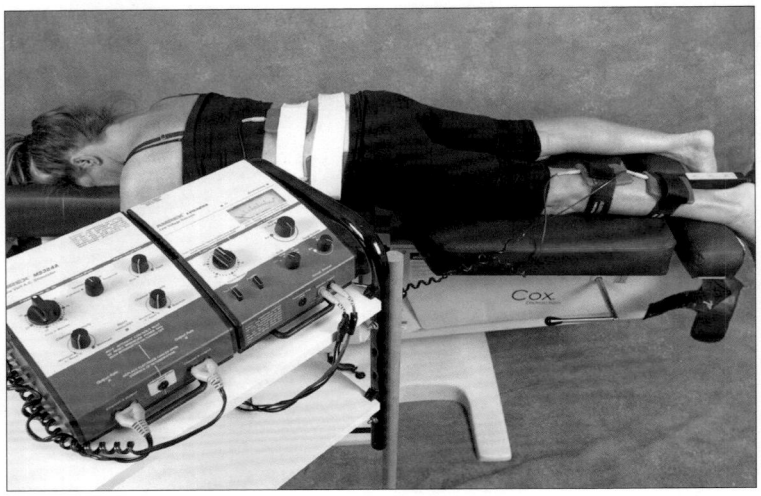

Figure 34
Physical therapy application

3. A belt support may be advised. This will prevent movement of the disc. It functions like a cast on a broken arm: prevent movement and allow healing.

4. Nutritional supplements may be advised to help heal the disc.

5. Kinesiology may be used. This is a balancing of the muscles in your low back and leg that is important in stabilizing weakness and problems of the low back.

6. Acupuncture or acupressure may be administered. "Trigger points" will be treated on the low back and extremities.

7. Exercises will be prescribed for you to do at home. These are to relieve pain and strengthen muscles.

*Although your physician may or may not use the specific treatment technique pictured and explained in this booklet, his/her goals remain the same: to help your understanding of your back condition, to guide you in controlling it, and to alleviate your pain.

General Instructions for Managing Low Back Pain:

IT TAKES THREE MONTHS FOR A HERNIATED DISC TO HEAL. ALTHOUGH THE PAIN MAY BE RELIEVED BEFORE THREE MONTHS OF CARE IS COMPLETED, THE DISC IS NOT YET HEALED TO ALLOW USUAL ACTIVITIES OF DAILY LIVING SUCH AS PROLONGED SITTING, BENDING, LIFTING AND TWISTING UNTIL THREE MONTHS' HEALING HAS TAKEN PLACE.

- A. **Do not sit!** Sitting increases the pressure in the disc up to 11 times higher than when you lie down. Therefore, in order to allow the disc to heal quickly and strongly, ***do not sit.***

- B. **Apply ice or heat as follows**: A) Apply ice for 20 to 30 minutes to the low back or buttock area as directed by the doctor. Or B) Alternate hot and cold to the low back and buttock—10 minutes of heat, then 10 minutes of cold, followed by 10 minutes of heat.

- C. **Rub analgesic liniment into the low back.** Massage liniment into painful areas after hot/cold therapy and/or the exercises.

- D. **Avoid constipation.** Straining at the stool can aggravate your low back and sciatic problems. If you are constipated, your doctor will prescribe something like Flax Plus Fiber to help.

- E. Take the following for healing of your back and leg problem:
    - ◊ Discat Plus—glucosamine sulfate/chondroitin sulfate/minerals — offers anti-inflammatory help and heals disc damaged tissue
    - ◊ Formula #2—bone-building formula for osteoporosis care and prevention
    - ◊ Formula One—enzyme, vitamin, mineral, herb, trace mineral formula for nutritional healing and immunity enhancement
    - ◊ Disc & Joint Pain Relief Complex—a natural pain reliever

- F. **Supplement your diet.** Most sciatic patients are given high doses of vitamins A, B, and C. Further, you are urged to eat a diet high in lean meat, vegetables, gelatin, fruits, fruit juices, especially grape, apple, and cranberry, and to avoid sweets, fried fatty foods, pork, carbonated and alcoholic drinks, and foods that constipate you. Increase your intake of fluids.

    Note: Your doctor may recommend a multiple supplement like Formula

One which provides nutritional factors for good health and immunity enhancement. For osteoporosis treatment and/or prevention, your doctor may recommend a non-phosphorous calcium supplement like Formula #2.

- ☐ G. **Be aware of sciatic pain's cycle.** It is important to realize the *seriousness of sciatic pain*. It is often discouraging when you start feeling better and then feel a pang of the old pain start back again. You will be told to expect this as *it is common to have recurrences during healing*. Avoid the movements that may aggravate your back: bending, lifting and twisting. Learn how to perform them properly.

- ☐ H. **Sleep on a good mattress.** Ask your doctor for a recommendation for a good, supporting mattress.

- ☐ I. **Sit in a good chair.** Sitting is an aggravator of back pain. Ask your doctor for a recommendation of a chair with proper contour.

- ☐ J. **Consider your job and its duties.** If your low back and leg pain condition is not so severe that the job won't irritate it, you will be allowed to work possibly. If your job entails sitting and bending of the spine which aggravate your condition, there is no choice but to have you avoid working until relief is attained. Discuss this with your doctor.

- ☐ K. **Exercise.** You will be asked to do exercises to ensure the relief of low back pain and sciatica as well as prevent its recurrence.

- ☐ L. **Appointments:** Keep them and be on time. We are committing to your healing; you must as well. Call if you must cancel, and re-schedule immediately.

- ☐ M. **Future Back Pain Episodes:** "Control, not cure" is often the motto in dealing with back pain. The combination of your vigilance in caring for your spine and our care is often appropriate. Should back pain ever return, consult with us then as well. We can help you again.